Connected Health: Technology-Enabled Care

Mbuso Mabuza

Published by Lekwandza Media, 2024.

CONNECTED HEALTH: TECHNOLOGY-ENABLED CARE

First edition. February 1, 2024.

ISBN: 979-8223495819

Written by Mbuso Mabuza.

Also by Mbuso Mabuza

A Healthy Mind And Best You: Achieving Great Results in Every Aspect of Your Life

Purposeful And Better You

Sustainable Development Calls for Effective Strategic Leadership for Efficient Health Systems

Health Promotion In Low Socioeconomic Settings

Medicine and Sociology of Health

Qualitative Methods In Public Health Research

Global Health Disaster Management

Global Health Policy And Programme Challenges

The Journey of Life Has a Gift of Purpose

Epidemiological Research

Ethics, Qualitative And Quantitative Methods In Public Health Research

When Love Lasts

Blockchain Technology In Healthcare And Medicine

Virtual and Augmented Reality in Healthcare

Data Analytics and Healthcare Informatics

How To Improve The Way You Think

Health Systems Engineering: Building A Better Healthcare Delivery System

Artificial Intelligence In Drug Discovery And Development

How To Make The Most Of Life

Precision Medicine

Connected Health: Technology-Enabled Care

Table of Contents

Preface

Connected health also known as technology-enabled care (TEC) is the collective term for telecare, telehealth, telemedicine, mHealth, digital health and eHealth services. Connected health involves the convergence of health technology, digital media and mobile devices. It enables patients, carers and healthcare professionals (HCPs) to access data and information more easily and improve the quality and outcomes of both health and social care.

Smart systems and infrastructures rely on mobile and pervasive technologies to offer end-users with portable and context-sensitive services that range from social networking, mobile commerce, to smart and connected health care. Considering service-driven computing for smart systems, the future of smart healthcare is hyper-connected, highly pervasive, and personalised. Mobile and pervasive technologies for mobile health (mHealth) and ubiquitous health (uHealth) systems provide a wide range of wellness and fitness applications as well as clinical and medical systems.

Mobile health or mHealth is a component of e-health (electronic health), and a medical and public health practice supported by mobile technology such as mobile devices and medical apps. Mobile health is poised to play a larger role in engaging patients in self-care as smartphone ownership is rising globally. Mobile health is a promising venue for reaching youth in general and may be particularly important for educating and addressing sensitive topics. Barriers such as privacy concerns and lack of integration into the electronic health record have limited the impact of apps, but mHealth has enormous potential to reshape healthcare delivery in the future.

Telemedicine may be considered as a component of virtual healthcare, since it involves the diagnosing and treatment of a patient, remotely. However, telemedicine specifically refers to the medicinal aspect of healthcare, whereby the clinician could use live audio-visuals and instant real-time messages to diagnose and treat a patient, remotely. Most people have unknowingly practised telemedicine when either seeking or giving medical advice over the telephone.

Nowadays, the nomenclature of telemedicine is created newly as "u-Health" in which ubiquitous technology is using to connect provider and patients in ubiquity. Technological system of u-Health will be easily established by convergence among ubiquitous and biometric technology, and mobile telecommunication infrastructure. However, the crucial point of the adoption and success of telemedicine in even ubiquity environments needs enough to tightly harmonise with the mainstream medicine.

TEC is capable of providing cost-effective solutions at a time when the demands on health and social care services continue to increase due to many countries' (especially high-income countries) growing and ageing population, the rising cost of advanced medical treatments, and severely constrained health and social care budgets. Indeed, wide scale adoption of TEC will be essential for sustaining the future health and social system.

The major areas of technical challenges in implementing TEC call for a focus on areas in need of change. mHealth appears to be testing the ability of our governments to confront the profound changes that mobile health technologies create. It is expected that interoperable global mHealth can produce meaningful improvement in the health of populations worldwide. Funding solutions are a necessary precursor to expanding mHealth and telemedicine to global delivery, and must be addressed in all planning, whether strategic or operational.

Chapter 1
Overview of Connected Health

Connected health also known as technology-enabled care (TEC) is the collective term for telecare, telehealth, telemedicine, mHealth, digital health and eHealth services. Connected health involves the convergence of health technology, digital media and mobile devices. It enables patients, carers and healthcare professionals (HCPs) to access data and information more easily and improve the quality and outcomes of both health and social care (Deloitte, 2015).

TEC is capable of providing cost-effective solutions at a time when the demands on health and social care services continue to increase due to many countries' (especially high-income countries) growing and ageing population, the rising cost of advanced medical treatments, and severely constrained health and social care budgets. Indeed, wide scale adoption of TEC will be essential for sustaining the future health and social system (Deloitte, 2015).

1.1 Telecare

TELECARE REFERS TO living independently in one's home with the application and help of ICTs. As well as assisting in the delivery of services, telecare maintains the security and safety of older people in their homes. There is a distinction between the two types of telecare systems: one is designed for assessment and information sharing, and the other is designed for management. However, the terminology shows that the above distinctions are grouped under two separate titles: risk management services as telecare; information sharing and assessment services as telehealth. The telehealth systems allow individuals with chronic conditions such as obstructive pulmonary disease (COPD), diabetes, heart failure or a mixture of these conditions to exchange data (e.g. blood levels) with healthcare professionals using a set of products such as blood pressure monitors, glucometers, and weighing scales. On the other hand, telecare systems focus on people who are constant need of health and social care services for support, and are facing difficulties carrying their current burden of responsibilities. Telecare technologies are a combination of wireless sensors and alarms that track the changes in an individual's activities and raise a call in the event of emergencies, such as fire or a fall. Personal alarms, temperature sensors, gas/water detectors, and bed occupancy sensors are only a few examples of the products that are used as a part of telecare services. The most important distinguishing factor between the two services is the matter of IS: the centralised and continuously monitored systems of telecare consist of more refined forms of information storage, retrieval, and filtering, and link to several actors responsible for care at once (Department of Health, 2009).

Telecare initiatives in search of more cost-effective ways of caring for older people and people with complex long-term conditions, have become a bigger part of some of the high-income countries' health agendas in recent years (Saunders et al, 2012). These services are more relied upon to bring major implications for health and social care services by transforming the order of care and extending the reach of healthcare outside of consulting rooms and hospitals (Oudshoorn, 2011).

⸻ ◉ ⸻

1.2 Telehealth

TELEHEALTH DESCRIBES healthcare delivery over distance or time using electronic communication technologies. It can be used to deliver essential care in resource-constrained settings and to distribute expertise that is usually concentrated to few centres. During the coronavirus disease 2019 (COVID-19) pandemic, telehealth visits also can address patient access issues by avoiding infection risks of in-person visits for older and immunocompromised at-risk patients. As described by Li et al (2020), a successful telehealth system requires an efficient, cost-effective data collection system with a centralised station for connectivity to multiple variable exposure and access to telehealth at different programs, a standardised curriculum that incorporates the best practices and key concepts would be essential. The key concepts in telehealth include the following:

- Honouring the doctor-patient relationship: Telehealth video visits, such as those using public-facing platforms, have the potential to strengthen the doctor-patient relationship because they are optimised for counselling, rather than data acquisition. Important but often neglected aspects of the clinical encounter, such as patient education, adherence to treatment recommendations, and assessment of activities of daily living, can be emphasised further through telemedicine visits. Furthermore, a virtual video telehealth visit can allow participation from several other family members, even if they live far from the patient.
- Billing and regulatory compliance: Trainees must understand the evolving billing and documentation regulations specific to telehealth. Additionally, licensure, security, and privacy regulations, although temporarily relaxed for the COVID-19 crisis, must be understood and followed.
- Integration of new technologies: Home monitoring for age-related macular degeneration. Curricula in telehealth should consider the role of new technology for at-home data acquisition.

- Promoting equity with telemedicine: A shift to increased tele-ophthalmology in the COVID-19 era can exacerbate disparities in access to care, especially in older adults or financially disadvantaged individuals who have low levels of health and technology literacy and those without access to broadband Internet. As clinicians, it is important to identify these barriers when setting up telehealth visits or programs and to promote resources that address issues related to Internet and technology literacy. Advocacy on behalf of these patients combined with proper use of telehealth eventually can lead to improvement in healthcare disparities because it allows patient outreach beyond a geographic practice catchment.

1.3 Telemedicine

IN SPITE OF NUMEROUS studies, unfortunately, there is no integrated definition of telemedicine. Telemedicine also referred to as telehealth or e-health describes the use of medical information exchanged from one site to another via electronic communications to improve the patients' health status. Although evolving, telemedicine is sometimes associated with a broader definition of remote health care services (National Academy of Sciences, 2012; Shirzadfar and Lofti, 2017).

The definition of the term telemedicine as accepted by the World Health Organization is, "The delivery of health care services, where distance is a critical factor, by all health care professionals using valid information and communication technologies for the exchange of valid information for diagnosis, treatment and prevention of disease and injuries, research and evaluation, and for the continuing education of health care providers, all in the interest of advancing the health of individuals and their communities" (Shirzadfar and Lofti, 2017).

Telemedicine, as one variety of digital health, is characterised by three criteria: using information and communication technology; covering a geographical distance; involving professionals who deliver care directly to a patient or group of patients. Technologies used include various types of ICT, like email, messaging systems, video communication systems, smartphones, tablets, wireless monitors, and other forms of telecommunication technologies. The main purposes comprise the provision of education (self-management support), exchange of information between healthcare providers (transfer of images and medical data), and facilitating contact with health professionals (continuous support from a distance). Telemedicine is said to facilitate access to relevant target groups and improve overall effectiveness of care (Timpel and Harst, 2020).

Telemedicine has a long rich history and a story that has not been told, certainly not in its entirety. The journey of telemedicine started with ancient societies and the early attempts to establish rudimentary communication connectivity between settlements when faced with internal or external threats and subsequently to establish clinical connectivity between patient and physician/caregiver/priest. Telemedicine provided the tools for connectivity when providers and recipients of care could not be in the same place and time (Seewon, 2010).

The origin of modern telemedicine applications can be traced in Europe and the fact that those by a Dutch physician, Willem Einthoven, had been by long distance transfer of electrocardiograms in 1905. After careful scrutiny, various sources can attest that the first clinical application in telemedicine was in cardiology, not radiology as some might have contended. This was followed by radio consultations from medical centres in Norway, Italy, and France in the 1920s, 1930s and 1940s for patients aboard ships at sea and on remote islands. The transmission of radiographic images began in the early 1950s in the United States of America, followed shortly thereafter by similar experimentation in Canada. The first wave of organised telemedicine programmes in the United States of America began in the late 1950s. It lasted nearly two decades and then came to a halt shortly after extramural funding was terminated. This was followed by a hiatus that lasted nearly a decade, until a new wave of telemedicine projects and programmes developed at a much larger scale than its forerunner. This last wave was led by state-based and province-based initiatives throughout the United States of America and Canada (Shirzadfar and Lofti, 2017; Seewon, 2010).

The deep roots of telemedicine are available in the archives of specialty areas in medicine (such as cardiology and radiology) and telecommunications and electronics is not necessarily available in the literature of telemedicine per se (Seewon, 2010).

In probing the history of telemedicine from the ancient to the present time, researchers discovered continuity and change existing side by side in a dynamic evolutionary process. Continuity stems from the convergence of medical care delivery and distance communication in various forms and manifestations, whereas change reflects the never-ending advances in the character and capability of the technology that enables telemedicine as well as other concurrent advances in medical science and medical practice (Seewon, 2010).

Nowadays, the nomenclature of telemedicine is created newly as "u-Health" in which ubiquitous technology is using to connect provider and patients in ubiquity. Technological system of u-Health will be easily established by convergence among ubiquitous and biometric technology, and mobile telecommunication infrastructure. However, the crucial point of the adoption and success of telemedicine in even ubiquity environments needs enough to tightly harmonise with the mainstream medicine (Seewon, 2010).

Telemedicine may be considered as a component of virtual healthcare, since it involves the diagnosing and treatment of a patient, remotely. However, telemedicine specifically refers to the medicinal aspect of healthcare, whereby the clinician could use live audio-visuals and instant real-time messages to diagnose and treat a patient, remotely. People's health can be monitored in their homes by devices that send information back to a central site by telephone or through the internet. Telemedicine can also be conducted by live interactive video-conferencing, with the patient seeing the doctor face to face, over a distance, with special devices used to assist clinical examination. Another form is store-and-forward telemedicine, where a photograph is taken of a skin lesion, for example, and attached to an email containing the relevant history, clinical findings and results of special investigations, and sent by a doctor or nurse to another doctor or specialist for diagnosis or second opinion. Most people have unknowingly practised telemedicine when either seeking or giving medical advice over the telephone (Mars and Erasmus, 2012).

According to the Institute of Medicine (1996), telemedicine is similar in most respects to other technologies for which better evidence of effectiveness is also being demanded. Telemedicine, however, has some special characteristics – shared with information technologies generally – that warrant particular notice from evaluators and decision makers. Most notably, telemedicine is not a single technology or discrete set of related technologies; it is, rather, a large and very heterogeneous collection of clinical practices, technologies, and organisational arrangements. In addition, widespread adoption of effective telemedicine applications depends on a complex, broadly distributed technical and human infrastructure that is only partly in place and is being profoundly affected by rapid changes in health care, information, communications systems.

The health problems of Africa are different from those of the developed world or old economies. Africa carries approximately 24 percent of the world's burden of disease, and is served by only 3 percent of the world's health workers, who have access to 1 percent of global health expenditure. Its population continues to grow rapidly and is expected to nearly double by 2050. As such, telemedicine holds great promise for Africa. It can provide rural healthcare in the most remote areas. All that is needed is a satellite or cellular communication link. This will reduce the long journey that people need to undertake, sometimes up to days on foot, to get to the nearest health care service point, like a clinic.

Telemedicine also increases access to scarce medical specialists in bigger centres and academic institutions. Through telemedicine, the geographic gap between colleagues is also overcome, as isolated doctors can receive support from their peers at a distance. The severe shortage of doctors can also be overcome by linking several health care facilities serviced by a health care worker to a doctor or doctors allocated to them.

Telemedicine provides a platform for delivery of education by leading minds in health and medicine to health workers and doctors in the field with minimum disruption to the delivery of health care services. Telemedicine also provides a platform for effectively facilitating research over a large geographic area in a short time (Mars and Erasmus, 2012).

Clinical telemedicine and informative telemedicine were defined by the World Health Organization (WHO) in 1998 as follows (Champ et al, 2015): "Clinical telemedicine is a professional activity that implements digital telecommunication facilities for physicians and other members of the medical profession to remotely perform medical procedures for patients." On the contrary, informative telemedicine is "an interactive audio-visual communication service that organises the dissemination of medical knowledge and protocols for patient care in order to support and improve medical activity." In other words, clinical telemedicine refers to the practice of distance medicine through technological means, while informative telemedicine concerns the dissemination of knowledge and information for medical use through the same means.

⸻⬥⸻

1.3.1 Informative telemedicine

INFORMATIVE TELEMEDICINE is defined as services that allow the remote delivery of medical information in order to improve medical knowledge and companies in charge of patients. This is the form of telemedicine developed in Northern Europe and North America, driven by the digital industry in the field of health and in legal terms of free access for members of the European Union (EU) to information society services (Andre, 2019). Its applications are the most widely used and shared with the electronic medical record (EMR) informative teleimaging and telemonitoring services for patients with chronic diseases.

Informative teleimaging

Informative teleradiology was not clinical at the beginning and dose not correspond at the moment to the good practices for radiologists. It consists of sending images via a transfer platform to a teleradiologist for a diagnostic remote interpretation, with little or no clinical information. The teleradiologist who practises on these platforms does not have the possibility to ask the requesting physician to obtain additional clinical information if he considers it necessary or to propose another type of imaging more appropriate to the question asked (Andre, 2019).

This practice of informative teleimaging is also developing in other medical specialties (dermatology, cardiology, ophthalmology, digestive endoscopy) with the help of algorithmic solutions of artificial intelligence (AI). AI applied to medical imaging will undoubtedly be an aid to medical diagnosis. The solutions proposed must be reliable, that is to say, of a sensitivity and specificity at least equal, if not superior, to human interpretation. These solutions must be validated by scientific studies published in peer-reviewed international journals (Andre, 2019).

In addition, the way in which the algorithm has been built must be transparent. The algorithmic solutions of AI must today make it possible to sort between a normal image and an abnormal image, that is to say, the capacity of the algorithmic solution to give a negative result toward a suspected anomaly, that is, a 100 percent specificity. The diagnostic sensitivity to an abnormal image will require human intervention for a long time. Deep learning solutions can advance the sensitivity of a diagnosis, such as screening for melanoma or diabetic retinopathy (Esteva et al, 2017; Rahimy, 2018). In summary, informative teleimaging will be able to rely more on AI to exclude an anomaly on condition that the specificity is 100 percent. This is the criterion generally used by the international health authorities that the marketing of AI solutions (FDA, CE marketing).

Remote telemonitoring

Another application of informative telemedicine is home telemonitoring services for patients with chronic diseases. This form of telemedicine is the major challenge of the transformation of health systems in the twenty-first century. The goal of these new healthcare organisations is to prevent aggravations of chronic diseases and hospitalisation. These new organisations in countries such as France combine clinical telemedicine and informative telemedicine.

The development of telemedicine services to monitor patients with chronic diseases is called for in all developed countries by the digital health industries. It is an important market creating many jobs.

Medical health professionals believe that the most successful chronic telemonitoring activities to date are those where the informative telemedicine service has taken into account the practices and organisations of health professionals. Projects initiated by health industry alone, without co0construction with medical health professionals, run the risk of failing.

For example, in France, the telecardiology program "remote monitoring of patients with an implanted defibrillator" has had an exemplary development, as it has been co-constructed with cardiologist. They regularly made improvements to the medical device and carried out medico-economic clinical studies, which led to the validation of the defibrillator implanted and connected by the High Authority for Health (Andre, 2019).

1.3.2 Clinical telemedicine

THE PRACTICE OF MEDICINE is an art, that is to say, a way of healing linked for a large part to the training received from practising masters who have built the exercise of this art on the acquired knowledge of medical science and their professional experience. In countries such as France, and many others, clinical teaching to future doctors is delivered to the patient's bed. Not all countries benefit from this training. In countries where the doctor's degree is obtained only after a university course of 5-6 years, new general practitioners or specialists must find placements, usually in hospitals, to apply the theoretical knowledge they have acquired, before exercising their art (Andre, 2019).

France and the many countries that have applied the model of clinical medicine have defined telemedicine as a form of remote medical practice that uses information technology (IT). The scope of practice of telemedicine is defined in France by law and an implementing decree for the conditions of implementation (Andre, 2019)

Teleconsultation

Tele-consultation may have several definitions depending on whether the country considers it as a clinical form of remote medical practice. It is thus necessary to distinguish between teleconsultation platforms that are informative telemedicine services and teleconsultation medical practices that are part of clinical telemedicine.

Two types of teleconsultation can be distinguished: the one programmed by the doctor and the immediate or unscheduled one requested by a person. The latter is often a personal medical e-consultancy (Simon, 2015).

Scheduled teleconsulation

Tele-consultation must take into account patients' rights to prior information so that consent can be obtained. This is the reason for recommending teleconsultation by the *Haute Autorite de Sante* (HAS) in France (Andre, 2019). Thus, to respect the deontological principles, a teleconsultaion cannot be done without a prior information of the persons concerned, in a fair, clear, and appropriate way, in order to collect their consent to this new medical practice. The teleconsultation can only be programmes, that is to say, it cannot replace a first consultation face to face, unless the interest of the patient justifies it. The programming of a teleconsultation makes it possible to provide access to the patient's computerised medical file if it has been opened by the patient. The file is essential for the doctor who performs a teleconsultation, especially in a person with chronic diseases that alternates face-to-face consultations and teleconsulations (Andre, 2019.

The practice of teleconsultation is not always well understood in relation to the traditional exercise of the medical art. This is a classic, face-to-face consultation that is conducted remotely by audiovisual communication means (Andre, 2019)

. When a doctor performs a classic consultation, he meets a person who considers himself sick. If it is a first appointment, it spends more time than when it is a follow-up consultation for a chronic disease. The first consultation necessarily involves a clinical examination, a prolonged interrogation on the personal and family antecedents, the treatments received, the surgeries carried out, etc. it includes an intellectual act that allows the physician to fully understand the subject of the complaint or request and to assess the health status of the new patient. Can a first consultation do as well? It is doubtful, because the climate of confidence that develops between the patient and his doctor during a first meeting is based on the warmth of a direct face-to-face relationship that cannot be reproduced by a first-time remote consultation by videoconference. In addition, it is exceptional that a first consultation does not require a clinical examination. All these points justify that the first consultation of a patient must take place face-to-face. It allows to inform and to obtain his consent when a follow-up by teleconsultation is proposed to him.

If it is not recommended when the person has easy and quick access to the doctor, a first teleconsultation may however be justified in certain circumstances, especially when the interest of the patient justifies it. This is the case in the acute phase of a stroke: the neurologist on duty in the neurovascular unit carries out a teleconsultation with the emergency department where the patient was received to judge the level of disability related to stroke and of the indication of thrombolysis after consulting brain imaging. This is also the case in the overseas regions for island populations: a first teleconsultation can be beneficial to judge the need or not to perform an evacuation by air ambulance. We can also think that for the prison population, the first teleconsultation is preferable to an extraction for a hospital consultation, if the state of the prisoner does not require a clinical examination (e.g., for a first consultation of psychiatry). Finally, a person with a severe disability and bed-ridden in a residential care facility, or in another institution, can benefit from a first teleconsultation to avoid a difficult and tiring journey (Salles, 2017). All these first consultations are done with the help of health professionals who are with the patient.

What would a patient think of a treating physician who during a face-to-face consultation would not bother to view the computerised medical record on their computer? Scheduled teleconsultation is indicated in a patient provided that the physician has access to his computerised record. This is a regulatory obligation for the physician. Teleconsulation between two face-to-face consultations is an added value in the follow-up of a patient with one or more chronic diseases because it allows a more regular follow-up without moving the patient. For example, teleconsultation at home is preferred by renal transplant patients. It prevents them from moving to the hospital and losing a day of work.

Immediate teleconsultation and personalised medical e-consultancy

Due to the initiative of private organisations (insurers, complementary health, other organisations), teleconsultation platforms have been developing for a few years now. This immediate access to a doctor is increasingly appreciated by urban workers who cannot find time to see their doctor or who do not want to wait for long hours in the emergency department. These new practices of immediate teleconsulation, followed sometimes by a tele-prescription, concern mainly benign affections. Such platforms are also developing in several European countries (the United Kingdom, Sweden, and Switzerland, among others).

Is this practice safe and secure for the patient and doctor? Opinion polls confirm the interest of these new practices since those interviewees estimate that 70 percent of the medical consultations can today be done by Internet without a physical examination. This possibility is of primary interest to parents with young children. To date, there is little scientific work to validate this immediate teleconsultation. In the event of a serious medical accident, the parents would not fail to turn against the doctor by reproaching him for failing to perform a physical examination. These teleconsultation platforms are more like medical e-consultancy platforms where the platform's doctor reassures, advises. Or directs according to his perception of the necessity and not of a face-to-face consultation with a physical examination.

The immediate medical e-consultancy (Simon, 2015) is a societal demand that has emerged for less than a decade, linked new ways of experiencing time and prioritising urgency and immediacy in all economic, social, and professional activities (Haute autorite de sante, 2018). The data revolution contributes to this evolution.

The personalised medical e-consultancy is considered in France as a legal practice of clinical telemedicine.

Is the personalised medical e-consultancy different from an immediate teleconsultation? This subject is under debate. It is important to distinguish these two practices for the following reasons. The personalised medical e-consultancy is based on information provided by the caller. This information is very fragmentary compared to that collected during a classic medical procedure where the doctor has the medical record and a clinical examination time. The medical e-consultancy cannot therefore, be assimilated to a consultation. Teleconsultation is also different from the medical e-consultancy because it is a generally programmed act that has been previously approved by the patient, clearly informed of the benefits and risks of this practice. In addition, teleconsultation, whether immediate or scheduled, must be done by video transmission, whereas most medical teleconferencing platforms are telephones. The personalised medical e-consultancy is not programmes, which does not allow the doctor to have sufficient and objective knowledge of the applicant's medical history. Thus, the personalised medical e-consultancy by Internet or by telephone platform cannot fulfil the ethical conditions of implementation of a teleconsultation.

The personalised medical e-consultancy has an interest in answering users' requests, in order to make a filter between what is an immediate medical consultation or a deferred consultation with the attending physician and what is possibly a real emergency not received by the appellant.

The practice of the personalised medical e-consultancy is not without risks for the doctor. She should not be paid on call but on vacation or salary. This form of fixed remuneration is found in European countries that have developed the medical e-consultancy (Sweden, the United Kingdom, Switzerland, etc.) the organiser of the platform must ensure compliance with regulatory requirements. The practice of telemedicine, in general, hardly lends itself to an acute or emergency situation, as a physical examination is usually necessary. This is the reason why most of the complementary mutual or insurance companies that manage these medical e-consultancy platforms immediately inform their members not to use them in case of emergency but to appeal to an emergency call centre.

When an attending physician is solicited over the phone by a member of his patient and gives him advice on a symptom or its treatment, he agrees to do so because he knows the medical record of the appellant and he thinks he can provide him with advice appropriate to his condition. In such a situation, the risk of medical error is not greater than a face-to-face consultation. The practice of telephone counselling, widespread in general practice, is generally downstream of a recent consultation and is somehow part of the same care. However, it is important for the doctor to make a phone call in the patient's medical file. It is different when a doctor practices the personalised medical e-consultancy for people he does not know.

The development of AI solutions could in the short or medium term modify the analysis that has just been done on the medical e-consultancy. These platforms held today by medical professionals or advanced practice nurses could be replaced by Chatbot robots. This solution is now being tested by the NHS in the United Kingdom (Burgeuss, 2017). Similarly, with the possibility of access to the medical records of a caller, the conditions for performing immediate teleconsultation could improve and integrate into a care path with the treating physicians, especially when they are inaccessible. Finally, solutions to help medical diagnosis by AI can only strengthen the safety and reliability of these new practices.

Teleexpertise

Teleexpertise is probably the telemedicine activity that will most structure new medical organisations in the twenty-first century. In fact, no doctor can today claim to possess a comprehensive knowledge of medical science to deal with health problems of a person as a whole. Over the years, medicine has reached a level of scientific complexity which partly explains the phenomenon of medical specialisations, or even overspecialisation, which has marked the last three decades.

Teleexpertise represents a new way of practising medicine (Simon, 2015). It enables medical professionals to consult each other regularly, to pool their medical knowledge, and to enhance their reciprocal competence. It only respects the doctor's ethical duties toward patients. Teleexpertise promotes the continuity of care and avoids the break that today represents too long appointment times in certain specialties. Direct teleexpertise between physicians, usually in the absence of the patient, can replace the specialised consultation and thus shorten the usual time for obtaining a specialised opinion. It allows the attending physician, coordinator of care, to ensure continuity of care in better conditions for the patient. This person must be informed of this practice and consent to it because it replaces certain specialised face-to-face consultations to which the patient, particularly the patient suffering from chronic illnesses, used to go and may wish to maintain. The patient must keep the free choice of the mode of specialised medical follow-up; that is why he must be informed of the possibility of this new practice, from which he can draw benefits in terms of continuity and quality of care. If the patient can oppose the teleexpertise, it is because he has been informed before. Consent should not be collected for each act of teleexpertise if the patient has initially agreed to the attending physician to this new form of care. He should be informed, however, that he can return to face-to-face consultations with the medical specialist if he is not satisfied. The patient may be attached to his specialist physician and may wish to have a face-to-face consultation from time to time.

The question of the tool used to carry out the teleexpertise is asked. The choice is the responsibility of the requesting physician who must comply with the telemedicine decree. If the attending general practitioner already has the practice of videoconferencing teleconsultation, the same tool can be used for programmed synchronous teleexpertise, provided that the requested specialist physician is himself equipped and available. Teleexpertise by telephone widely practised in recent years, is no longer recommended as it will cause failure of the requesting doctor and the doctor asked to remember to ensure the traceability of information given and received in the patient's medical file. Such negligence would be blamed on the doctor if his responsibility was implicated in a medical accident of a patient who had benefited from a teleexpertise by telephone. Realising a teleexpertise with the same equipment and protocols devolved to teleconsultation puts the doctor away from such risk.

Asynchronous teleexpertise by secure messaging in health is the recommended form of teleexpertise that will be the most commonly practised in the short term. It allows the secure transfer of medical pictures, such as skin picture, EKG, etc., and confidential clinical information in writing. So, the answer of teleexpet physician can integrate the medical record. The situations of the teleexpertise practice are numerous (Simon, 2015).

Teleexpertise in primary care is used to avoid the patient to move in classic consultation with the medical specialist. The attending physician directly consults his specialist colleague on the basis of elements in the medical file. This way of working is demanded by the new generation of general practitioners who, during their internship, have made the habit of consulting their hospital colleagues about their patients. Young doctors are destabilised when they arrive on the ground of the liberal exercise and they no longer have the opportunity to seek specialist advice almost immediately as in the hospital. In primary care, quickly obtaining such advice facilitates the coordination of care and avoids a break in continuity of care. The young doctors understood that telemedicine made it possible to do otherwise than to ask patients to make their own appointment with the specialist with waiting times of several months. Teleexpertise with the specialist saves time, enhances the role of the attending physician, and strengthens interprofessional cooperation. In addition, the pooling of knowledge between general practitioners and medical specialists has the advantage of mutually enhancing skills. It is the learning function of telemedicine.

The practice of regular, even daily, teleexpertise between public or private health facilities is an inevitable organisational evolution to improve the care path of patients in a health territory or region. As demonstrated by the study of the Midi-Pyrenees region conducted in the 1990s (Simon, 2015), the practice of inter-institutional teleexpertise makes it possible to better manage the hospitalisation of a patient and to avoid, once in two, an unnecessary transfer to the referral hospital or university hospital. It allows emergency services to avoid certain hospitalisations, especially those requested for specialised advice.

The success of a teleexpertise practice makes it necessary to review the medical organisations whatever the place of exercise. In the hospital sector, medical specialists in the reference establishment must integrate into their daily practices a time offer of service to the small establishments of the territory.

In the outpatient sector, the demand for specialised expertise also needs to be organised differently. Multi-professional healthcare home are the primary care structures that have most anticipated these developments. They will benefit from the organisations set up in the health establishments. It is also important that the liberal specialists organise themselves to offer primary care physicians their teleexpertise service.

Second-opinion teleexpertise was one of the first applications of telemedicine in radiology. Radiologists distinguish telediagnosis as "the exploitation of the transmission of images for the remote obtaining of a primary and definitive diagnosis, in the absence, from the patient of a radiologist to interpret these images immediately." The absence of a radiologist from the patient justifies that telediagnosis is assimilated to a teleconsultation, the teleradiologist having the possibility, if he deems necessary, to interrogate the patient remotely. The assimilation of telediagnosis to a radiological teleconsultation has been recognised in France in the latest teleradiology charter. Radiological teleexpertise differs from telediagnosis; it is a second opinion given to the requesting radiologist by a more expert radiologist. For radiology departments, the expert radiologist authorised to give a second opinion must meet at least two of the following criteria: the recognition by professionals of their organ specialty, an important daily practice in various pathologies within its domain expertise, a minimum number of files seen per year, participation in staff and multidisciplinary consultation meetings, and possibly research and teaching activities in the field concerned. In addition, the expert radiologist must practise in relation to or belong to a centre of competence or reference (Societe Francaise de Radiologie, 2009).

The permanence of teleradiology care at the level of a territory, or even a region, is of two natures. When the establishment of a given territory does not have a radiologist to the patient, it is the radiologist of the reference institution, or even a private radiologist company, who provides a teleconsultation for the interpretation of the examination. This requires that the radiological examination rooms be equipped with videoconferencing systems to enable the teleradiologist required to interrogate the patient if necessary and that a regional or national digital platform can promote image transfers, their accommodation, and telemedicine practices between institutions.

In the field of pathology, telepathology practices between experts have developed in recent years, at the regional, national, or even international level. It is most often second-opinion teleexpertise, sometimes enriched with diagnostic interpretation by AI algorithms (Alami et al, 2017; Maxman, 2018). It is in the field of telepathology that teleexpertise could be assimilated to a telediagnosis.

Teleexpertise is now remunerated in France under the common law of Social Security. This act of telemedicine is not recognised in all countries and is sometimes considered a teleconsultation. It is developing rapidly in low- and middle-income countries that are beginning the epidemiological transition to chronic diseases of ageing. The use of teleexpertise at a national or even international level in these countries, particularly in sub-Saharan Africa, makes it possible to compensate for the shortage of specialist doctors (Diby et al, 2017).

1.4 Mobile Health (mHealth)

SMART SYSTEMS AND INFRASTRUCTURES rely on mobile and pervasive technologies to offer end-users with portable and context-sensitive services that range from social networking, mobile commerce, to smart and connected health care. Considering service-driven computing for smart systems, the future of smart healthcare is hyper-connected, highly pervasive, and personalised. Mobile and pervasive technologies for mobile health (mHealth) and ubiquitous health (uHealth) systems provide a wide range of wellness and fitness applications as well as clinical and medical systems (Iwaya, Ahmad and Babar, 2020).

There are various definitions of mobile health or mHealth. For example, mHealth has been defined as mobile computing, medical sensor, and communication technologies for healthcare (Park, 2016). The World Health Organization defines mobile health or mHealth as a component of e-health (electronic health), and a medical and public health practice supported by mobile technology such as mobile devices and medical apps (Oracle Health Sciences, 2017).

Increasingly, mHealth is emerging from the early adopter phase and is transforming many aspects of the healthcare and medical industry and can even be applied to understand the effects and reliability of data within clinical trials by using dosing algorithms and making data available to the investigators through the use of devices such as sensors and wearables.

Mobile health is poised to play a larger role in engaging patients in self-care as smartphone ownership is rising globally. Mobile health is a promising venue for reaching youth in general and may be particularly important for educating and addressing sensitive topics. Growing evidence supports the use of mobile applications (apps) as an acceptable and often preferred way for teens to receive sexual health information and to successfully engage at-risk youth. The Monsenso mHealth solution can help healthcare providers to closely monitor patients who have experienced a first episode of mental illness. The Monsenso mHealth platform includes a triple-loop treatment model that connects patients, family and carers and care providers. The solution is configured to support the treatment of most mental illnesses and it can also be configured to meet specific clinical needs. Advances in smartphone software and hardware coupled with rising availability of wearable devices have resulted in exponential growth in the health apps market. Barriers such as privacy concerns and lack of integration into the electronic health record have limited the impact of apps, but mHealth has enormous potential to reshape healthcare delivery in the future (Paul et al, 2021; Monsenso, n.d.).

Despite emerging evidence supporting mHealth efficacy (such as for improving health outcomes), some individuals have concerns about mHealth technology that may impede scalability, efficacy, and, ultimately, the public health benefits of mHealth. There are features of mHealth that lead to worries about the potential negative effects on an individual's health (such as due to exposure to electromagnetic and radio waves), despite evidence supporting the safety of these technologies. This may represent an important implementation barrier and may also have broader ramifications (Materia, Faasse and Smyth, 2020).

Mobile health (mHealth) approaches that use mobile phones in support of health care can help overcome some of the barriers associated with clinic-based care. Mobile phones are ubiquitous in both developing and developed countries, even among people with serious mental illness, who often have limited access to resources. Research across continents has shown that the majority of adults with serious mental illness are interested in using their mobile phones as instruments for self-management. Early mHealth efforts have produced promising outcomes in terms of feasibility, acceptability, and preliminary efficacy in this population. Whether mHealth interventions can serve as stand-alone treatments, effectively engage with serious mental illness in remote care, and produce clinical outcomes that are comparable to those of clinic-based interventions are made accessible in real-world practice, patients and their providers will have more options to choose from when deciding on their preferred model of care. Direct comparison of the strengths and weaknesses of existing interventions for a designated clinical problem is at the core of comparative effectiveness research (Ben-Zeev et al, 2018).

mHealth applications that are sensitive to the user needs of vulnerable populations have the potential to gain uptake in more diverse communities. Consideration to the visual and linguistic design of mHealth applications along with how mHealth applications are introduced to patients in their health-related needs and address social determinants of health, to promote greater usage and understanding of health applications, although this has not been studied (Liu et al, 2020).

———◉———

1.5 Digital health and eHealth services

DIGITAL HEALTH IS AN umbrella label for a wide range of technologies that could meet the healthcare challenges of the present consumer-driven era. Digital health tools refer to the technologies that deliver services to consumers and patients and help them manage personal health and wellness.

Digital health technologies use computing platforms, connectivity, software, and sensors for health care and related uses. These technologies span a wide range of uses, from applications in general wellness to applications as a medical device. They include technologies intended for use as a medical product, as companion diagnostics, or as an adjunct to other medical products (devices, drugs, and biologics). They may also be used to develop or study medical products.

The following areas are commonly understood as being part of, or related to, digital health: mobile health (mHealth), wearable devices, telehealth, telemedicine, personalised medicine, artificial intelligence, big data, blockchain, health data, health information systems, the infodemic, the Internet of Things, and Interoperability.

Digital technologies are now integral to daily life, and the world's population has never been more interconnected. Innovation, particularly in the digital sphere, is happening at unprecedented scale. Even so, its application to improve the health of populations remains largely untapped, and there is immense scope for use of digital health solutions.

The World Health Organization is harnessing the power of digital technologies and health innovation to accelerate global attainment of health and wellbeing. The Global Strategy on Digital Health adopted by the World Health Assembly, presents a roadmap of concrete actions to leverage the foundational and cutting-edge developments in digital health, and catalyse their use among member states in order to improve health outcomes. The purpose of the World Health Organization's Global Strategy on Digital Health is to support all countries in strengthening their health systems using digital health technologies and to achieve the vision of health for all. The Strategy is designed to be fit for purpose and for use by all Member States, including those with limited access to digital technologies, gods and services (World Health Organization, 2021).

eHealth, "the use of information and communication technologies for heath, first arose in health care in the form of electronic health records (EHRs). These electronic records are data-rich sources that go beyond clinical management of patients and can also be used to improve quality performance in health care organizations and contribute to medical research efforts. eHealth is a means to provide high-quality care for an increasing number of people and to do so cost-effectively and efficiently. eHealth tools include products, systems and services that go beyond simply Internet-based applications.

Chapter 2

Impact of Mobile Health (mHealth) and Telemedicine

The impact of mobile health and telemedicine encompasses the following domains to be used as a measurement framework: access to care, financial impact/cost, experience, and effectiveness, in the context of Africa, Asia, Europe, North America, and South America.

Telemedicine, the practice of using telecommunications technology to augment local clinical care, can be a significant part of the solution to improving rural health. At its core is a central hub, staffed by experienced nurses, family medicine experts and other specialists. By telephone, internet and data transfers, these skilled professionals could link with general practitioners at rural outposts (McKinsey & Company, 2011).

mHealth is used by most countries as a tool to improve healthcare access by eliminating the geographic barriers from the healthcare equation. In other jurisdictions it is seen as a way to improve the poverty situation of people in rural communities (Nsor-Anabia, Udunwa and Malathi, 2019).

Put in practice, mobile health (mhealth) and telemedicine can improve access to healthcare for patients in rural areas, improve the quality of care and reduce costs.

2.1 Africa and Asia

IN EGYPT, IT IS AN advantage that there is availability of international funding schemes (e.g. European Union, United States of

American aid) (Hussein and Khalifa, 2012). Utilising the Egyptian Cloud Computing Centre of Excellence to launch telemedicine applications as services; incorporating many initiatives for eHealth open source applications; the social networks (Facebook, twitter, etc.) can be highly utilised in the social awareness programmes (Hussein and Khalifa, 2012).

Opportunities for telemedicine are that many governmental initiatives for information and communication technology literacy such as the Information Technology Clubs (Hussein and Khalifa, 2012). Telemedicine could be a part of the eGovernment (Hussein and Khalifa, 2012).

Telemedicine business models and initiatives taken by the private sector, mainly mobile operators present opportunities for adoption in healthcare and medicine in countries such as Egypt (Hussein and Khalifa, 2012).

There are several strengths of telemedicine. No cultural or social barriers towards information and communication technology utilisation (internet, mobile technologies) (Hussein and Khalifa, 2012). It is an advantage for telemedicine that there is a cheap cost service provided at the governmental healthcare enterprises in Egypt (Hussein and Khalifa, 2012).

It is a strength that the Ministries of Health have established regulatory bodies in countries such as Ethiopia. Utilising the eHealth programmes undertaken by the Ministry of Communication and Information Technology and the Ministry of Health for capacity building and applications development (Hussein and Khalifa, 2012).

Much as there are strengths, there are also weaknesses of telemedicine. Fears of losing certain jobs when eHealth system will be deployed. Unavailability of the advanced medical devices incorporated in TeleHealth networks in the Egyptian market, is a challenge. Other challenges for telemedicine are that there are no laws of eHealth practice; no regulatory framework for information security, privacy and safety.

Lack of adopting the international industrial standards for interoperability. Lack of benchmarking and evaluation schemes for telemedicine (Hussein and Khalifa, 2012).

Threats include the old generations or the ageing population relatively resisting the automation process. Limited support from the government; no sustainable business models for telemedicine. Lack of stakeholders' commitment to take responsibilities in utilising telemedicine according to the regulations. No strategies for implementing eHealth at the national scale and no commitment to adopt telemedicine (Hussein and Khalifa, 2012).

In terms of mHealth, the Measure SMS-Morbidity tool can be used with different approaches to obtain patient estimates. Using the data sent through SMS, a lymphatic filariasis programme is able to map prevalence of clinical disease and identity priority areas in need of managing morbidity and prevention of disability interventions (Mableson et al, 2017).

Two-tier reporting mechanisms will reduce the number of people that need to be trained in SMS reporting, as data collectors will only need to be trained in the identification of lymphatic filariasis clinical conditions and only data reporters trained on sending the SMS. Implementing a two-tier reporting system such as the high endemic, urban, two-tier reporting scenario in Tanzania, and the high endemic, rural, two-tie reporting scenario in Nepal, reduces the burden of the survey on healthcare services by sharing the workload of data collection and reporting between health workers (Mableson et al, 2017).

House-to-house census methods used in highly endemic areas provide an accurate estimate of patient numbers in implementation units which enables countries to effectively plan and target resources equitably. However, in low endemic implementation units, in which low patient numbers are anticipated, it is important to have a more cost-effective implementation scenario. In highly endemic implementation units in which high numbers of patients are anticipated, this method may lead to under-reporting which may lead to inadequate levels of care being planned and provided. While the scenarios have been developed based on experiences in African and Asian lymphatic filariasis programmes, application of Measure SMS-Morbidity is not limited to the scenarios from Bangladesh, Ethiopia, Malawi, Nepal and Tanzania (Mableson et al, 2017).

Short message service-based mobile telephone intervention could indeed improve the effectiveness of frontline HEWs in rural Ethiopia, primarily in the area of improving access to antenatal care, delivery services, and postnatal care. No significant impact was observed in the rate of contraceptive utilisation and immunisation coverage. It is recommended that systematic awareness programme on the potential mHealth on health for the concerned stakeholders be initiated (Atnafu, Otto and Herbst, 2017).

In highly endemic implementation units in which high numbers of patients are anticipated, the application of Measure SMS-Morbidity method may lead to under-reporting which may lead to inadequate levels of care being planned and provided (Mableson et al, 2017).

⸻ ◉ ⸻

2.2 Europe

DIVERSIFYING FUNDING schemes and increasing commitment from the telemedicine industry; promoting multi-source financing and public-private partnerships in funding; and reviewing existing incentives presents opportunities for telemedicine in the European Union (European Commission, 2018). Good prospects for telemedicine trade, and that this could bring benefits to importing" countries in terms of cost-savings and faster delivery of care and to exporting" countries in the form of foreign exchange and quality improvement (Alvarez, Chanda, and Smith, 2011).

There is a dedicated budget from the European Commission to telemedicine projects, and national or regional funding mechanisms promoting sustainability of initiatives within the European Union. Cost-effectiveness of telemedicine within the European Union is a strength (European Commission, 2018).

However, there are limited resources for set-up and ongoing operation of telemedicine services, especially in underserved settings (Wootton, Jebamani and Dow, 2005). Financial constraints were a common barrier and challenge for telemedicine implementation in countries such as Maldives (Nazviya and Kodukula, 2011).

Limited financial support from governments within the European Union is a weakness for adopting telemedicine (European Commission, 2018). There is increased workload for healthcare professionals if data coexists with paper; "Silo thinking" and lack of cooperation between primary and secondary care; Enduring strong national focus from telemedicine market players; Market players fear a potential loss of intellectual property (European Commission, 2018).

Inappropriate use of existing resources could potentially deter future investment in telemedicine (Wootton, Jebamani and Dow, 2005). Financial burden of initial investment in telemedicine; expensive solutions from some market players in the context of the European Union (European Commission, 2018).

Complexity of relationship and interest management between the various players and stakeholders, and interoperability challenges to European Union fragmentation poses a risk for the adoption of telemedicine (European Commission, 2018).

The common barriers and challenges for telemedicine implementation in Maldives were identified to be financial constraints, limitation of technological infrastructure, limitation of human resource capacity in the rural areas, lack of public awareness and community sensitisation on telemedicine, limitation of trust within the health system, limitation of commitment from politicians, limitation of commitment from other stakeholders and limitations on the legislative support for telemedicine (Nazviya and Kodukula, 2011).

In low-endemic implementation units, in which low patient numbers are anticipated, application of Measure SMS-Morbidity can be costly, and, as such, it is important to have a more cost-effective implementation scenario (Mableson et al, 2017).

The still low digital literacy of the public, in particular, the over-65-year old users, for high-income countries such as Italy, explains the scarce offer of mHealth products to favour self-management of chronic diseases such as diabetes mellitus (Rossi and Bigi, 2017). In other settings, it is viewed as an advantage that patient awareness is changing expectation about mHealth applications. Generally, the younger generations are mobile technology savvy, and, as such, implementation of mHealth applications is perceived to be easily adopted among the new generations. By contrast, other observers see no correlation between being mobile technology savvy and adoption of mHealth interventions regardless of age, sex, or ethnic origin. An interesting observation is that interventions such as mHealth applications should not be implemented as a blanket approach, but the uniqueness of each setting should be taken into consideration (Mabuza, 2018; Mabuza and Shumba, 2018).

Regulators are grappling with issues about what constitutes a mobile device and the boundary between a mobile device and the communication infrastructure it uses. This can be viewed as a contrasting dichotomy whereby the regulation of the healthcare and medical industry puts emphasis on protecting the public, guided by the principle of 'first do no harm', whereas the regulation of the communication industry places emphasis on fostering competition (Vos, n.d.). It is worrying that there is ambiguous liability as there is no case law or no indication of who will be liable if things go wrong with mHealth applications. Even if there were to be globally applicable regulations for mHealth, such regulations would fall short because it is not possible to rationalise as different countries or regions require different formulas.

Decrease in patient travel for health services among underserved populations (Wootton, Jebamani and Dow, 2005). Overall high digital literacy of the population in high-income countries such as within the European Union (European Commission, 2018).

Lack of public awareness and community sensitisation on telemedicine, limitation of trust within the health system and limitation of commitment from other stakeholders were among the common barriers and challenges for telemedicine implementation in countries such as Maldives (Nazviya and Kodukula, 2011). Fear of malpractice among healthcare providers, and lack of patient/social awareness of telemedicine among countries within the European Union (European Commission, 2018). Low income per capita affects access to telemedicine networks (internet, iPhone, etc.); no national coverage of the medical insurance (Hussein and Khalifa, 2012). No clear and efficient reimbursement models within the European Union (European Commission, 2018).

It is an opportunity that the new generation of physicians and patients is very eager to utilise the new technologies (Hussein and Khalifa, 2012). There are opportunities to develop proper dissemination and communication strategies to overcome medical doctors' reluctance on implementation of telemedicine within the European Union. It is an opportunity that new generations or young people are more comfortable with using technologies in healthcare within the European Union. Use of already interested public and private stakeholders as levers to increase acceptance of telemedicine is an opportunity for countries within the European Union. Communication with the public of countries within the European Union can increase awareness of how important open data and data sharing are, pertaining to the implementation of telemedicine (European Commission, 2018). There is an opportunity to develop telemedicine new reimbursement frameworks for countries within the European Union (European Commission, 2018).

Some of the challenges include possible reluctance of the population to use telemedicine services, especially among underserved settings. Many of the world's most marginalised populations lack access to technologies, and even among those that have such access, there may be lack of ability to use technologies. At a more basic level, communities with low levels of literacy will automatically be excluded from text-based communication technologies such as email. Another threat to telemedicine is the possible reluctance of health professionals to deliver telemedicine services (Wootton, Jebamani and Dow, 2005).

Other threats include loss of the doctor-patient relationship and of the social link; the elderly's resistance of technology in the care process; and lack of experts' commitment to telemedicine practices (European Commission, 2018). Lack of coordination between European Union countries in establishing reimbursement rules is also a threat (European Commission, 2018).

There is need for national policy/strategy in telemedicine, and policy focus on chronic disease management among countries within the European Union (European Commission, 2018).

Limitation of commitment from politicians, and limitations on the legislative support for telemedicine can be a hindrance for the implementation of telemedicine applications in countries such as Maldives (Nazviya and Kodukula, 2011).

Regulatory and policy weaknesses of implementing telemedicine in the European Union include legal loopholes regarding liability and data confidentiality and security; poor regulatory framework, lack of standards and guidelines; misalignment of national policies might jeopardise regional-wide or global-wide uniform approach to telemedicine; and different data privacy policies (European Commission, 2018).

A lack of medicolegal protocols for Telemedicine services among underserved populations, is a challenge (Wootton, Jebamani and Dow, 2005). Persisting lack of interoperability between solutions and difficulty in aligning national standards and protocols; different political priorities and interests hindering the wider use of telemedicine (European Commission, 2018).

It is true that diabetes is a disease affecting more seriously low-income levels of society worldwide, and, as such, the mHealth tools to favour self-management and adherence should be available to the larger public for free. For the Italian market, the scarce offer of products might be partly explained by the still low digital literacy of the Italian public, in particular, the over-65-year old users. In order to have mHealth applications with a stronger impact on user's critical thinking skills as is requested for the aim of self-management, the design of mHealth devices should be based on solid theoretical models of education and communication (Rossi and Bigi, 2017).

Achieving a minimum level of cross-linked knowledge of all involved parties may facilitate wider use of telemedicine solutions among member states of the European Union; increased motivation for education and training in telemedicine; multiply health technology assessments to obtain a systematic evaluation of properties, effects and impacts of telemedicine intra-country and inter-country within the European Union; greater involvement of European Union health technology assessments bodies recently that are able to provide scientific-based evidence for member states of the European Union and beyond (European Commission, 2018).

Insufficient interoperability; poor system reliability and response time are a challenge within the European Union. There is also the risk of technological flaws; risk of data leaks; data overload can create resistance; different technological levels and advancement of involved national bodies and stakeholders (European Commission, 2018).

2.3 North America

PARK ET AL (2018) OBSERVED that the use of telehealth increased dramatically in the period 2013-2016 across all population groups in the United States of America. Rates of consumers' use of telehealth by type of use in decreasing order were communication by phone, asking medical questions through email, making online appointments, viewing test results through a website, communicating by a mobile app, communicating by live video, communicating by text message on a mobile phone, communicating by live text chat on a website, respectively. While there was evidence that populations with limited mobility were among the highest users, key underserved populations had significantly lower use of telehealth. This suggests that state efforts alone to remove barriers to using telehealth might not be sufficient for increasing use, and new incentives for both providers and consumers to adopt and use telehealth may be needed.

Overall, there are five major areas of technical challenges in implementing mHealth: usability; system integration; data security and privacy; network access; and reliability. These challenges call for a focus on areas in need of change: identification of storage locations when cloud computing is in use; usability analysis of mHealth applications and improvements made based on this usability analysis; considering HL7 standards for interoperability; and reliability analysis of mHealth applications before use (Gurupur and Wan, 2017).

Canadian mHealth regulation is overseen by Health Canada (HC). HC and federal and provincial governments rely on non-profit, government-funded organisations, such as the Canadian Agency for Drugs and Technologies in Health (CADTH), to provide evidence, research and analysis and set non-binding regulatory standards to assist with decision-making around healthcare technology regulation and to adopt new digital technologies within healthcare systems (Jogova, Shaw and Jamieson, 2019).

Two major challenges to mHealth regulation and adoption emerge in HC's existing regulations: Canada lacks a specific regulatory framework for mHealth; lack of clarity in what guidance is available, which provide little in the way of consolidated, comprehensive, easily understandable guidance for app manufacturers who may not be well-versed in legal or regulatory language. Both challenges are associated with further concerns (Jogova, Shaw and Jamieson, 2019).

For Canada to become a leader in mHealth, it must look to the regulatory steps taken by the United States of America, the current innovator in this field, to develop its own devoted guidelines that strike a balance between protecting users and promoting innovation. It must also actively engage in nascent multinational regulatory efforts, as neither the regulation of this border-traversing technology nor the realisation of its benefits with checks on its risks can feasibly be achieved in isolation. Regulation can ultimately benefit businesses by adopting standards that would reduce barriers to market entry, stimulate innovation, reduce user risk, enable product export and encourage adherence to regulations (Jogova, Shaw and Jamieson, 2019).

⸺⸺◉⸺⸺

2.4 South America

LATIN AMERICA HAS WITNESSED gradual improvements in its health indicators. Yet, amid these improvements disparities remain, with health outcomes in rural areas lagging those in urban areas. The challenge behind closing this healthcare gap is unique. Suboptimal health outcomes in rural Latin America are tied to limited availability of medical knowledge in these areas, which manifests itself as less well-trained primary care physicians and the relative absence of specialists.

In Brazil, for example, primary care physicians in the rural regions often lack opportunities for continuing education and there are no performance-based incentive systems to encourage self-improvement. In addition, clinics in rural regions are often staffed by less-qualified doctors, those who cannot find jobs in the cities, or by inexperienced, young doctors waiting to be accepted into urban residency programmes. The relative absence of specialty care physicians in rural areas is related to insufficient local demand, generally unattractive living conditions and a lack of opportunities for advancement (McKinsey & Company, 2011).

Taken together, these factors lead to limited access to healthcare, as shown by long waiting lists for referrals; low quality care; higher costs than necessary. It is estimated that more than 120 million people are affected across Latin America, about a fifth of the region's population (McKinsey & Company, 2011).

From a practical standpoint, the three barriers that have blocked rapid expansion of telemedicine services have been largely overcome:

- **Medical knowledge** has advanced significantly, and, for most conditions, diagnosis and treatment are straightforward for competent practitioners or specialist. This is especially true for ailments common in rural areas.
- **Remote evaluations** are easier to conduct with technological advances bringing a plethora of low-cost devices to the market. These instruments, for instance, can transmit electrocardiograms to a central hub for immediate evaluation.
- **Communication** is no longer a limiting factor in many rural areas as mobile telephone and internet access has become widespread.

The more intransigent obstacle centres on local skills. Limited availability of managerial skills is the most significant factor preventing governments from deploying telemedicine more aggressively. Countries that have successfully created a telemedicine system have addressed the need for managerial skills by building partnerships with private-sector players. MedicalHome, a Mexican for-profit joint venture with telecommunications company TelMex, provides 24-hour medical services to a million families. Unlike the telemedicine model in Brazil, MedicalHome works directly with patients, who are encouraged to contact the central hub with their concerns. Patients are assisted according to evidence-based protocols developed by the Cleveland Clinic. MedicalHome operates on a flat $5-a-month subscription model (McKinsey & Company, 2011).

Increased use of telemedicine in South America can lead to improved health and longer lives in the hard-to-reach rural regions. A programme in Brazil shows that advances in technology, medicine and communication have made expanded deployment possible. Now, governments must work with the private sector to make it reality (McKinsey & Company, 2011).

Analysing the successes in Mexico and the lessons learned in Brazil, there are three core responsibilities that governments should assume to boost telemedicine. These measures focus on bringing in private-sector partners who can add managerial discipline and creativity to the system. First, governments must provide a supportive ecosystem, allowing remote treatment decisions while ensuring quality standards. Next, governments must map out clearly their priorities for telemedicine. Lastly, governments should seek private-sector suppliers able to address these priorities effectively (McKinsey & Company, 2011).

Improving healthcare in rural Latin America requires bringing medical knowledge and expertise to hard-to-reach areas. Telemedicine can achieve this goal. Medical practices, technology and communications have advanced far enough that they are no longer substantial obstacles to deploying telemedicine systems. The final hurdle is gathering appropriate managerial skills around the efforts. By partnering with private-sector providers, governments can harness their skill and reach the full potential of telemedicine (McKinsey & Company, 2011).

Alvarez, Chanda, and Smith (2011) observe that there are good prospects for telemedicine trade, and that this could bring benefits to "importing" countries in terms of cost-savings and faster delivery of care and to "exporting" countries in the form of foreign exchange and quality improvement. However, there were some concerns regarding quality of care, regulation, accreditation and data security. As such, countries may wish to consider entering bi-lateral agreements, as they provide more potential to address the concerns and capitalise on the benefits. More data should be collected, both from the volume of telemedicine trade and on the impact it is having on health systems, as currently there is very limited data on this.

2.5 Conclusion

INFORMATION AND COMMUNICATION technologies have great potential to address some of the challenges faced by both developed and developing countries in providing accessible, cost-effective, high-quality health care services. Telemedicine uses information and communication technologies to overcome geographical barriers, and increase access to health care services. This is particularly beneficial for rural and underserved communities in developing countries – groups that traditionally suffer from lack of access to health care (World Health Organization, 2010).

Different types of telemedicine services like store and forward, real-time and remote or self-monitoring provides various educational, healthcare delivery and management, disease screening and disaster management services all over the globe. Even though telemedicine cannot be a solution to all the problems, it can surely help decrease the burden of the healthcare system to a large extent (Chellaiyan, Nirupama and Taneja, 2019).

The importance of satellite communications is emphasised in the field of disaster management when all terrestrial modes of communication are disrupted. International telemedicine initiatives are bringing the world closer and distance is no longer a barrier in attainment of quality healthcare. Now, telemedicine services can be made available to all irrespective of time, place, social status, race or gender (Chellaiyan, Nirupama and Taneja, 2019).

While low- and middle-income countries are more likely to consider resource issues such as high costs, underdeveloped infrastructure, and lack of technical expertise to be barriers to telemedicine, high-income countries are more likely to consider legal issues surrounding patient privacy and confidentiality, competing health system priorities, and a perceived lack of demand to be barriers to telemedicine implementation. It is recommended that both developed and developing countries can take steps to capitalise on the potential of information and communication technologies including telemedicine or telehealth. One such step is creation of national agencies to coordinate telemedicine and eHealth initiatives, ensuring they are appropriate to local contexts, cost-effective, consistently evaluated, and adequately funded as part of integrated health service delivery. Ultimately, telemedicine initiatives should strengthen – rather than compete with – other health services (World Health Organization, 2010).

The importance of evaluation within the field of telemedicine cannot be overstated: the field is in its infancy and while its promise is great, evaluation van ensure maximisation of benefit. Information and communication technologies can be costly, as can be the programmes using them to improve health outcomes. Indeed, the most frequently cited barrier to the implementation of telemedicine solutions globally is the perception that the cost of telemedicine is too high. Closely linked to cost is cost-effectiveness (World Health Organization, 2010).

While there was evidence that populations with limited mobility were among the highest users of telemedicine in the United States of

America, key underserved populations had significantly lower use of telemedicine or telehealth. This suggests that state efforts alone to remove barriers to using telemedicine or telehealth might not be sufficient for increasing use, and new incentives for both providers and consumers to adopt and use telemedicine or telehealth may be needed (Park et al, 2018).

Much as there are good prospects for the use of telemedicine, there are some concerns regarding quality of care, regulation, accreditation and data security. As such, countries may wish to consider entering bi-lateral agreements, as they provide more potential to address the concerns and capitalise on the benefits. More data should be collected, both from the volume of telemedicine trade, and, on the impact, it is having on health systems, as currently there is very limited data on this (Alvarez, Chanda, and Smith, 2011).

What is needed now is a telemedicine awareness campaign among health workers especially in developing economies such as in Africa, and international support for low-bandwidth clinical telemedicine across borders. It will require international effort to resolve issues related to licencing and liability. Furthermore, one should not lose sight of the necessary skills to manage and maintain the technology that enables the successful functioning of telemedicine (Mars and Erasmus, 2012).

There is an opportunity as new legislation can be the foundation of wider use of telemedicine among countries within the European Union. Finding common ground between European Union Member States' legislations and national standards' and defining clear rules on liability when using telemedicine solutions. Restrictive (privacy) laws might hinder data sharing (European Commission, 2018).

Even though the mHealth sub-sector is relatively young, it is transforming the health delivery ecosystem around the world, and more so around the low- and middle-income economies where concrete benefits such as increased accessibility and associated information, especially in remote geographies are recorded. There is also a rise in diagnostic ability and disease tracking, prompt and quick action on health matters as well as magnified access to medical training and education for health professionals which have been corroborated mHealth (Nsor-Anabia, Udunwa and Malathi, 2019).

There are many pros and cons to using mobile technology in the healthcare and medical field. The advantages of using mobile equipment are that smartphones allow practitioners to complete tasks in remote locations. For example, a physician can use their smart phone or tablet to access a patient's EHR, review medical histories, allowing them to send text message alerts about payment schedules and outstanding bills. Mobile communication can also cut down on snail mail, paper use, and time spent on phone calls. Mobile apps give professionals, administrators and patients, greater flexibility. They are an inexpensive way for facilities to provide more high-quality services, and – at the same time – are cheaper for patients to access. Some generate better health awareness, while others assist communication between patient and care providers.

Here are some of the areas that 'mhealth' apps can assist with: chronic care management, medication management, medical reference, diagnostics, personal health records, women's health, fitness and weight-loss, mental health. The disadvantages of mobile technology in healthcare and medicine are that even with advanced technology, human error cannot be erased completely. Mobile devices can be easily lost or stolen. Smart phones and tablets are also vulnerable to hacking, malware, and viruses – especially if the devices are used on unsecured internet connections. mHealth systems face significant challenges related to data security and privacy that must be addressed to increase the pervasiveness of such systems (Iwaya, Ahmad and Babar, 2020).

mHealth is used by most countries as a tool to improve healthcare access by eliminating the geographic barriers from the healthcare equation. In other jurisdictions it is seen as a way to improve the poverty situation of people in rural communities. However, technological challenges, illiteracy, sociocultural difficulties and finances are among the serious obstacles to a successful implementation of the intervention (Nsor-Anabia, Udunwa and Malathi, 2019).

It is recommended that systematic awareness programme on the potential mHealth on health for the concerned stakeholders be initiated (Atnafu, Otto and Herbst, 2017). In order to have mHealth applications with a stronger impact on user's critical thinking skills as is requested for the aim of self-management, the design of mHealth devices should be based on solid theoretical models of education and communication (Rossi and Bigi, 2017).

The major areas of technical challenges in implementing mHealth call for a focus on areas in need of change: identification of storage locations when cloud computing is in use; usability analysis of mHealth applications and improvements made based on this usability analysis; considering HL7 standards for interoperability; and reliability analysis of mHealth applications before use (Gurupur and Wan, 2017).

mHealth appears to be testing the ability of our governments to confront the profound changes that mobile health technologies create. Similar to developed nations, developing countries confront mHealth policy issues related to data security, licensure, and patient confidentiality and privacy that represent major obstacles. Because extant international best practices may be inappropriate for furnishing adequate guidance for these countries, there is the potential of formulating practices that are specific to developing nations. However, doing so could result in a two-tiered system of best practices that may fuel divisions between developed and developing nations (Malvey and Slovensky, 2017).

It is expected that interoperable global mHealth can produce meaningful improvement in the health of populations worldwide. Policy formulation, which is inherently challenging, is more complex when multiple states or nations seek to achieve a common goal despite their disparities. Evidence suggests that governments can impede or facilitate global policy, and resulting bureaucracies can also impede private sector initiatives, even those with substantial financial investment capability. Strong, credible policy advocates are needed to initiate local efforts that can be leveraged to build more extensive partnerships and collaboratives to address the persistent problem of folding mHealth as a delivery model. Funding solutions are a necessary precursor to expanding mHealth to global delivery, and must be addressed in all planning, whether strategic or operational (Malvey and Slovensky, 2017).

Bringing mHealth interventions to scale requires input from a number of stakeholders, especially community and implementers, from the initial planning to the dissemination of the intervention. mHealth platforms need to be easily adaptable and developers must have a view to implementation in all stages of the development process. Rapid adaptation during scale-up taking into account contextual differences allows for more broad dissemination. Public health policymakers and funders must see the value in the mHealth approach and be committed to enact policy and health systems changes that enhance the feasibility and sustainability of the intervention (Paul et al, 2021).

mHealth applications that are sensitive to the user needs of vulnerable populations have the potential to gain uptake in more diverse communities. Consideration to the visual and linguistic design of mHealth applications, along with how mHealth applications are introduced to patients, may increase adoption and acceptability (Liu et al, 2020).

The first concern associated with the lack of a specific regulatory framework for mHealth is the financial and opportunity costs of app development which shows evidence of the financial barrier to market entry. Second, traditional methods of medical device evaluation to establish safety and efficacy are costly and time intensive and assume that the approved device is relatively static. Although this may work for medical equipment, apps are often updated every few weeks, cost little and may function differently on different hardware platforms. This poses a challenge to clinical assessment and to establishing the version of, and platform for, the app being evaluated, particularly as regulations apply to the app and not its associated device. Third, is the issue of data security; because app manufacturers and private businesses fall outside the scope of health information legislation. This oversight must be addressed if healthcare providers are to use this technology for patient care. Current regulations incentivise mHealth manufacturers to create apps that do not require regulation, leading to a proliferation of health and fitness apps rather than software directed at complex healthcare challenges (Jogova, Shaw and Jamieson, 2019).

mHealth appears to be testing the ability of our governments to confront the profound changes that mobile health technologies create. Similar to developed nations, developing countries confront mHealth policy issues related to data security, licensure, and patient confidentiality and privacy that represent major obstacles. Because extant international best practices may be inappropriate for furnishing adequate guidance for these countries, there is the potential of formulating practices that are specific to developing nations. However, doing so could result in a two-tiered system of best practices that may fuel divisions between developed and developing nations (Malvey and Slovensky, 2017).

It is expected that interoperable global mHealth can produce meaningful improvement in the health of populations worldwide. Policy formulation, which is inherently challenging, is more complex when multiple states or nations seek to achieve a common goal despite their disparities. Evidence suggests that governments can impede or facilitate global policy, and resulting bureaucracies can also impede private sector initiatives, even those with substantial financial investment capability. Strong, credible policy advocates are needed to initiate local efforts that can be leveraged to build more extensive partnerships and collaboratives to address the persistent problem of folding mHealth as a delivery model. Funding solutions are a necessary precursor to expanding mHealth to global delivery, and must be addressed in all planning, whether strategic or operational (Malvey and Slovensky, 2017).

Chapter 3

Future Perspective of Mobile Health (mHealth) and Telemedicine

As with any disruptive healthcare innovation, it takes time, validation, and the right catalyst before it becomes fully embraced across the medical community. With the coronavirus pandemic, one innovation is at the forefront of transforming the healthcare landscape – telemedicine (Modern Healthcare, 2021).

To illustrate the impact telemedicine will make in the future (reshaping the future healthcare landscape), the following are some of the predictions healthcare leaders and telemedicine providers from multiple specialties provided when asked about how they anticipate telemedicine reshaping the future healthcare landscape (Modern Healthcare, 2021):

- Telemedicine will become a standard service offered across all care settings
- Patients will choose providers, health systems, and hospitals based on telemedicine access.
- Medical facilities that embrace telemedicine will see business and revenue growth
- Telemedicine will become an efficient option for preventative care
- Access to specialists will become the norm, which will benefit hospital wait times

The use of telemedicine increased substantially during the COVID-19 pandemic. As the pandemic continues and evolves, it will be important to continue to monitor the level of telemedicine use as well as expectations regarding post-pandemic use levels. As the practice of physicians will evolve to integrate an increasing number of elements of virtual care, it is of utmost importance to prepare the workforce for this evolution (Grossman et al, 2020).

Although the future is bright, more research is needed to determine optimal ways to integrate telemedicine – especially remote monitoring – into routine clinical care. Policy changes are needed to overcome regulatory and reimbursement challenges (Serper and Volk, 2018).

mHealth is set to expand rapidly over the next decade, driven by and building on the successes seen in key therapy areas such as cardiac rhythm management. Further impetus will be given by the expansion of M2M technologies and the rise of the Internet of Things. As the opportunities mHealth offers to patients, healthcare providers and funders are realised, business cases will strengthen, leading to over more new projects in a self-reinforcing cycle. No one stakeholder will be able to drive success; this will be achieved through partnerships between a ranges of participants. New mobile technologies will continually enhance the potential and possible uses of mHealth, as they emerge. Medical apps and other mHealth systems will enable people's health to be monitored much more closely and accurately in the very near future: So, people with long-term conditions will be able to go back to work, where previously they might have had to stay at home or in hospital (Vodafone, 2015).

Apps are changing the health and social care industry. The ubiquitous smartphone has found its way into the pockets of nearly every clinician, care provider and patient in recent years, and, by 2030, the development and integration of apps will have helped transform the way services are delivered. By 2030, apps will have reached a mainstream position sitting alongside traditional support services, having established a solid evidence of reducing healthcare costs, improving the efficiency of care delivery and enabling greater access to high-quality care via telemedicine. mHealth will be prescribed, seen as an everyday toolkit that patients use alongside or instead of drugs. Self-management with remote monitoring via health app will be as acceptable to a patient or care provider as traditional methods of care delivery are today. The patient will be central to the success or failure of apps. In the future, only apps that meet a true need for the consumer will thrive. Another big change that is anticipated is that apps will be aggregated. That is, there will be a move from the silos we see today, to an ecosystem of data. This will enable clinicians to access one picture, pulling information from a variety of apps into one dashboard. This extends the personalised, integrated, whole life proposition that apps will offer (ORCHA, n.d.).

mHealth initiatives are being increasingly tested to improve health care delivery in developing countries such as India, among others. there needs to be highlighted the poor quality of the current evidence base and an urgent need for focused research aimed at generating high-quality evidence on the efficacy, user acceptability, and cost-effectiveness of mHealth interventions aimed toward health systems strengthening. A pragmatic approach would be to include an implementation research component into the existing and proposed digital health initiatives to support the generation of evidence for health systems strengthening on strategically important outcomes (Bassi et al, 2018).

The barriers (such as governance and risk management, trust and safety, systems and process, awareness and habit, return on investment) faced by the industry will each be overcome over the next decade. Governments will set the bar for standards, with a clear process for applying the criteria and an active programme to raise awareness amongst professionals and consumers. This will be accompanied by a drive to educate the workforce with training and education, in order to change the culture and sentiment towards mHealth. A concerning barrier is physicians' resistance to change, and their reticence to adopting technology in care delivery. More will need to be done to ensure appropriate digital training for clinicians, or a "knowledge gap" will grow between current and future staff (ORCHA, n.d.).

There is good reason to be excited over mHealth. Mobile technology can enable much-needed, thoroughgoing change in healthcare systems worldwide and in turn bring significant social and economic benefits. The scope of the task ahead, though, should temper the current excitement. The adoption of mHealth, if it is to be meaningful, must be part of a wider disruption of healthcare. But however ripe the sector is for change, the barriers remain substantial. Powerful stakeholders with contradictory incentives will either fail to underwrite change that benefits the system as a whole but not themselves, or use the complexities of systems to block innovation that might harm them. Disruption is never easy, but is rarely impossible. Already mHealth is being adopted where the need is greatest and the barriers are lowest: among those who pay a large proportion of income for healthcare, among patients who are not getting effective care from existing structures and, most of all, in emerging markets. Ultimately, mHealth will probably become commonplace as to fade from notice. In several years the bits of mHealth that work won't be called 'mHealth': they will be called 'health', in the way that nobody talks about 'electric health' and no country has a 'stethoscope society'. mHealth will have reached its full potential when it becomes ordinary (PwC, 2014a).

References

Alami, H. et al. (2017) The challenges of a complex and innovative telehealth project: a qualitative evaluation of the eastern Quebec telepathology network. *Int J Health Policy Manag*, 7(5), 421-432.

Alvarez, M.M., Chanda, R. & Smith, R.D. (2011) How is telemedicine perceived? A qualitative study of perspectives from the UK and India. *Globalization and Health*, 7:17.

Andre, A. (2019) *Digital medicine*. Springer.

Atnafu, A., Otto, K. & Herbst, C.H. (2017) The role of mHealth intervention on maternal and child health service delivery: findings from a randomised controlled field trial in rural Ethiopia. *mHealth*, 3:39.

Ben-Zeev, D. et al. (2018) Mobile health (mHealth) versus clinic-based group intervention for people with serious mental illness: a randomised controlled trial. *Psychiatric Services*, 69, pp. 978-985.

Burguess, M. (2017) *The NHS is trialing an AI chatbot to answer your medical questions*. Wired, 5 Jan.

Champ, S.P. (2015) et enjeux de la telemedicine, 17-19, in *Telemedecine – Enjeux et pratiques*, Collection Syntheses et reperes, Le Coudrier Editions, Brignais, octobre, 190 p.

Chellaiyan, Nirupama, A.Y. & Taneja, N. (2019) Telemedicine in India: where do we stand? *Journal of Family Medicine and Primary Care*, 8, pp. 1872-1876.

Diby, F. et al. (2017) Connaissances, attitudes et pratiques des professionnels de la sante face aux opportubites de diagnostic et de prise en charge des pathologies cardiovascularies par la telemedicine en Cote d'Ivoire. *Eur Res Telemed*, 6, 35-42.

Esteva, A. et al. (2017) DEermatologist-level classification of skin cancer with deep neural networks. *Nature*, 542(7639), 115-118.

European Commission (2018) Market study on telemedicine.

Gurupur, V.P. & Wan, T.T. (2017) Challenges in implementing mHealth interventions: a technical perspective. *mHealth*, 3:32.

Haute autorite de sante (2018) *Qualite et securite des actes de teleconsultation et de teleexoertise.* Avril.

Hussein, I.and Khalifa, I. (2012) Telemedicine in Egypt: SWOT analysis and future trends. *GMS Medizinische Informatik, Biometrie und Eoidemiologie,* 8 (1).

Institute of Medicine (1996) *Telemedicine: a guide to assessing telecommunications for health care.* IOM.

Iwaya, L.H., Ahmad, A. & Babar, M.A. (2020) Security and privacy for mhealth and uhealth systems: a systematic mapping study. *IEEE Access,* X.

Jogova, J.S., Shaw, J. & Jamieson, T. (2019) The regulatory challenge of mobile health: lessons for Canada. *Healthcare Policy,* 14(3), pp. 19-28.

Li, J-PO, et al. (2020) Digital telemedicine and artificial intelligence in ophthalmology: a global perspective. *Progr Retin Eye Res,* Sep 6:100900.

Liu, P. et al. (2020) Use of mobile health applications in low-income populations. *Circ Cardiovasc Qual Outcomes,* 13:e007031.

Mableson, H.F. et al. (2017) Community-based field implementation scenarios of a short message service reporting tool for lymphatic filariasis case estimates in Africa and Asia. *mHealth,* 3:28.

Mabuza, M. (2018) Impact of an onsite occupational health clinic on organisational performance and employee wellbeing at a southern African maritime port. *Eurasian Journal of Medicine and Oncology,* 2(3), 152-164.

Mabuza, M.P. & Shumba, C. (2018) A qualitative exploration of doctors and nurses' experiences on the management of TB and HIV coinfection in a TB-HIV high burden community in northern KwaZulu-Natal, South Africa. *Journal of Public Health in Africa,* 9(1), 19-24.

Malvey, D.M. & Slovensky, D.J. (2017) Global mHealth policy arena: status check and future directions. mHealth, 3:41.

Mars, M. & Erasmus, L. (2012) *Telemedicine can lower health care costs in Africa.* Innovative.

Materia, F.T., Faasse, K. and Smyth, J.M. (2020) Understanding and preventing health concerns about emerging mobile health technologies. *JMIR MHealth and UHealth*, 8(5):e14375.

Maxmen, A. (2018) Deep leraning sharpens views of cells and genes. *Nature*, 553(7686), 9-10.

McKinsey & Company (2011) Perspectives on healthcare in Latin America: from quantity to quality: the health of the Brazilian healthcare system.

Monsenso (n.d.) mHealth – the future of mental health care.

National Academy of Sciences (2012) *The role of telehealth in an evolving health care environment.* The National Academic Press: Washington.

Nazviya, M & Kodukula, S. (2011) Evaluation of critical success factors for telemedicine implementation. *International Journal of Computer Applications*, 12 (10), 29-36.

Nsor-Anabia, S., Udunwa, U. & Malathi, S. (2019) Review of the prospects and challenges of mhealth implementation in developing countries. *International Journal of Applied Engineering Research*, 14(12), pp. 2897-2903.

Oracle Health Sciences (2017) mHealth and the transformation of clinical trials: harnessing data advanced analytics and the internet of things to optimize digitalized clinical trials. Oracle White Paper, June 2017.

Park, J. et al. (2018) Are state telehealth policies associated with the use of telehealth services among underserved populations? *Health Affairs*, 37 (12), 2060-2068.

Park, Y. (2016) Emerging new era of mobile health technologies. *Health Informatics Research*, 22(4), pp. 253-254.

Paul, M.E. et al. (2021) Scale up mhealth HIV interventions: site and public health perspectives and lessons learned from P3. *mHealth*, 7:38.

Rahimy, E. (2018) Deep learning applications in ophthalmology. *Curr Opin Ophthalmol*, 29(3), 254-260.

Rosi, M.G. & Bigi, S. (2017) mHealth for diabetes support: a systematic review of apps available on the Italian market. *mHealth*, 3:16.

Salles, N. (2017) *Telemedecine en EHPAD, les cles ppour se lancer.* Ed. Le Coudrier, 69530 Brignais; octobre.

Seewon, R. (2010) History of telemedicine: evolution, context, and transformation. *Health Informatics Research*, 16(1), pp. 65-66.

Shirzadfar, H. & Lofti, F. (2017) The evolution and transformation of telemedicine. *International Journal of Biosensors & Bioelectronics*, 3(4), pp. 303-306.

Simon, P. (2015) Les differents actes de telemedicine, 77-108, in *Telemedecine – Eneux pratiques*, Collection Syntheses et reperes, Le Coudrier Editions, Brignais, octobre, 190 p.

Societe Francaise de Radiologie (2009) *Charte de la teleradiologie.* Sept.

Timpel, P. & Harst, L. (2020) Research implications for future telemedicine studies and innovations in diabetes and hypertension – a mixed methods study. *Nutrients*, 12(1340).

Vos, J. (n.d.) *Policy and regulation for innovation in mobile health.* PA Consulting Group.

Wootton, R., Jebamani, L.S. & Dow, A. (2005) E-health and the Universitas 21 organization: telemedicine and underserved population. *Journal of Telemedicine and Telecare*, 11, 221-224.

World Health Organization (2010) *Telemedicine: opportunities and developments in member states.* Report on the second global survey on ehealth. Global Observatory for eHealth Series – Volume 2.

Letter from the author

Dear Readers, Bloggers, Podcasters, Youtubers and Book Reviewers

Reading is a great way to personal growth, inspiration and healing. I was touched by a story of a man who read books during his mourning period following the death of his wife and children due to a car accident. I was also touched by a story of a woman who also read books during her chemotherapy treatment because it helped her to take her mind off her unpleasant procedure. A month before she was diagnosed with cancer, that particular woman had also lost her beloved mother who succumbed to a terminal illness. Through her unwavering faith, she firmly believed that "life is a gift" in spite of what she had been through.

Very recently, during the COVID-19 pandemic, I was touched by the story of a woman who was a trailblazer, a pioneer, a shining business leader, a hands-on coach, and a revolutionary consultant who had shared business advice with many aspiring entrepreneurs in Africa for over a decade. When you read through it all, know that this is a message of hope. It is a message meant for you. If you find time, read it until the end. The woman was suffering from a rare form of cancer. The doctors could not do anything for her.

Her body had collapsed, and she felt she was closer to death, and she knew it. Her body was in severe pain, and sleeping was an ordeal. She was also too weak and ill to do anything really. She could not meet friends, she could not talk much on the phone. She had no energy to watch movies, write, walk, or play. Now add to that she was a single mom, and had the sole responsibility for her young children. Now add to this, that the businesses she had built over the last ten years were hanging on a thread after many months of her absence. And in this ultra-vulnerable time, she lost her friend, the one who gave her strength throughout. And just when she made some progress in her recovery and she thought 'the story of loss' was complete ... she suddenly lost her sweet mom. Her mom was buried in her absence, because she was simply too weak to travel and attend her funeral.

All of that ... in a matter of ten months. She had lost plenty. Death and loss were her new comrades. Sometimes, life has other plans for us. She knew that many people in this world go through much worse, but here is her story ... and what she learnt from it.

"Here is what I want to let you know ... I have not figured it all out – far from it ... But I know this: Loss is a part of life. When you resist what you have lost, you suffer. When you embrace it and seek life's lessons and your soul's essence in your pain, you will find plenty of GIFTS in your agony. And you know you will be fine. Yes, I have lost tremendously over the last ten months. And in very profound ways. But instead, I decided each day to focus on what I have received: I have received a new and very caring guardian angel (my mom). I received the immense joy of watching the birds, the sun, the trees, and the clouds in my garden every single day.

I received the caring kindness of friends, and family, and complete strangers. I received the ability to understand my body and mind in a way most people and doctors would never be able to [well, not many people get to sit with it for over 300 days straight]. I am filled with immense gratitude for my children, my father, the surrounding peace, my clients and online community (you!), my team, and the past version of myself who built a sanctuary of a home in Africa.

I no longer fear death or separation. I received a new perspective of life ... So much so that the huge pains and deaths I have experienced resulted not in suffering ... but in a level of appreciation, gratitude, love, inner abundance, and peace I have never experienced before. Beyond my pain, I found a more peaceful and authentic version of me.

Hence, I learnt that ... Your suffering is not created as a result of your hardships. Instead, your suffering is created by the perspective of your mind when you face hardship. Our SOUL, however, knows instinctively how to handle it. Let me remind you that most of the things you worry or stress about each day: They – do – not – matter. Let go of it.

All will fall into place when the time is ripe. Do not go down the spiral of stress, worry, anger, or sleeplessness nights ... be it in regard to your money issues, people you deeply love, people who hurt you or who do not understand you, actions you regret, challenging situations, an unclear future, slow progress, your illness, injustice, or personal loss. It will only weaken you profoundly from the inside out. As a result, you sabotage your inner power ...You bury the energy that makes you feel ALIVE ... And you dim the light of your soul's wisdom.

How did I overcome huge loss and pain at all levels? I actively sought the connection with my higher self, nature, and the spiritual world. And told myself the story of abundance and healing over and over again until it felt real. I smiled often.

We live in very challenging times. In many ways, I and many of you ... are a victim of that.

Hence, I want to remind you that it is more important than ever that we focus on what really matters.

Replenish your inner strength in the face of challenge. Find it. Nourish it. You will need it.

Focus on your dreams, your virtues, and whatever makes you smile. Appreciate your blessings (because you are surrounded by plenty) ...

Seek comfort and healing in Mother Nature and the spiritual world ... as they are packed with signs, answers, and wonders ...

Be who you TRULY are. UNAPOLOGETICALLY.

And let no one and nothing take away your unique power, your inner peace, and your smile.

Maybe that is the true freedom so many of us are longing for?"

Because of this, I put a sample of the book *How To Make The Most Of Life*' at the back of this book.

My hope is that my journey in writing will find my books in the hands of readers all over the world and touch hearts for the better.

Life has showed me that there is so much more to writing. The wonderful thing is that I have discovered a world of wonderful people with either a love of reading, writing, or both, so willing to share their opinions and be a catalyst to my writing.

Reviews are a tremendous influence online, and it would really help me reach my writing goal if you would please write a quick review of this book through your chosen online bookstore or platform. Your feedback tells me what you want to see more or less of. I believe we never stop learning. It is a lifelong gift to grow and change.

I invite you to join the mailing list to stay informed of all the new upcoming promotions and book give-aways.

Much love,

Mbuso Mabuza (Dr)

mbusoprecio@gmail.com

Don't miss out!

Visit the website below and you can sign up to receive emails whenever Mbuso Mabuza publishes a new book. There's no charge and no obligation.

https://books2read.com/r/B-A-JPJL-TRRLC

BOOKS 2 READ

Connecting independent readers to independent writers.

Did you love *Connected Health: Technology-Enabled Care*? Then you should read *Precision Medicine*[1] by Mbuso Mabuza!

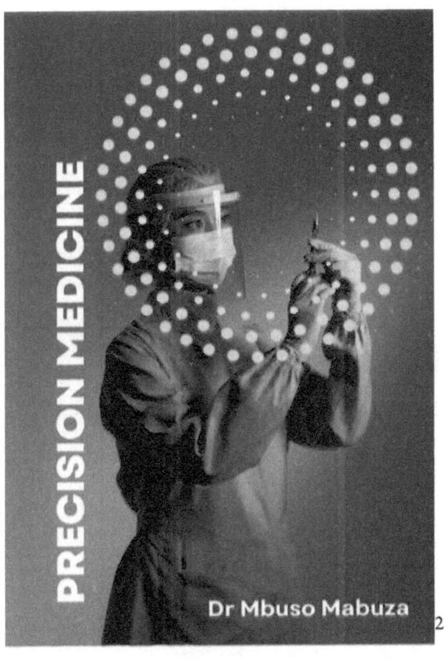

[2]

With the present emerging artificial intelligence (AI) technologies, computational "machine learning" techniques for training and generalisation from data, and cutting-edge statistical techniques, will play a significant role in analysing multidimensional datasets generated by the new technologies of systems medicine. This progressively but rapidly leads to a "new taxonomy," generating new approaches for disease diagnosis, therapy, and clinical decisions, promising more individualised treatments and improved outcomes for patients. Indeed, if this approach becomes efficient in clinical practice, it provides a real paradigm change in health care, from reactive to proactive medicine.

---

1. https://books2read.com/u/4NgErJ

2. https://books2read.com/u/4NgErJ

Precision medicine will allow big data patterns to emerge and algorithms to be developed, which, in turn, will allow more predictive and precise decisions about one's health to be made. Considering the rapid scientific advances in genomics and the vast adaptation of wearable technology and other quantified self-applications, it is likely only a matter of time before this data will play a larger and more integrated role in public healthcare services.

Precision medicine, sometimes called personalised medicine, is an emerging technological advancement which aims to personalise prevention and treatment according to the genetic, environmental, and lifestyle variability of individual persons or a specific group of people with commonalities, as opposed to the 'one-glove-fits-all' approach which has less consideration for the uniqueness of the individual person or specific group of people with commonalities such as similar genetic changes in a tumour.

Perhaps, the clearest utility of precision medicine approaches thus far has emerged from efforts to improve disease diagnosis with the promise of better treatment. This perspective emerged as a critique of medical practices characterised as employing reductionist and oversimplified methods of disease categorisation.

Treatment is not the only aim of precision medicine, but prevention is also important as genetic testing for people with a family history of a certain illness such as diabetes mellitus, could also receive tailored preventive measures before those people even get sick. As such, precision or personalised medicine is driven not only by individual health data, but also by the availability of reference medical knowledge and evidence, that is, precision or personalised medicine is linking knowledge with individual health data for decision support.

The current evolution of personalised medicine is happening at a fast pace, whereby it goes beyond therapeutics selection for a patient but into the realm of drug discovery, planning and delivery of care, and engagement between consumers and companies focusing on the improvement of healthcare. Such rapid evolution of personalised medicine is largely driven by advances in diagnostics, digitalisation, data and analytics operating across a broad scope.

Nonetheless, precision or personalised medicine can be considered as the cornerstone of modern medicine. With so many hospital admissions being attributed to a 'one-size-fits-all' prescribing approach and adverse drug reactions being among the leading causes of death globally, not to mention the huge economic implications this creates, a tailored approach for every patient is needed. At the centre of this should be pharmacogenomics with the goal to improve drug safety and efficacy. Furthermore, therapy for each patient should be designed according to their personal characteristics, health status, lifestyle and pharmacogenetic profile. Ultimately, the goal of precision or personalised medicine is to contribute towards preventive, predictive and participatory health systems.

Also by Mbuso Mabuza

A Healthy Mind And Best You: Achieving Great Results in Every Aspect of Your Life
Purposeful And Better You
Sustainable Development Calls for Effective Strategic Leadership for Efficient Health Systems
Health Promotion In Low Socioeconomic Settings
Medicine and Sociology of Health
Qualitative Methods In Public Health Research
Global Health Disaster Management
Global Health Policy And Programme Challenges
The Journey of Life Has a Gift of Purpose
Epidemiological Research
Ethics, Qualitative And Quantitative Methods In Public Health Research
When Love Lasts
Blockchain Technology In Healthcare And Medicine
Virtual and Augmented Reality in Healthcare
Data Analytics and Healthcare Informatics
How To Improve The Way You Think
Health Systems Engineering: Building A Better Healthcare Delivery System
Artificial Intelligence In Drug Discovery And Development
How To Make The Most Of Life
Precision Medicine
Connected Health: Technology-Enabled Care

About the Author

Dr Mbuso Mabuza is a highly motivated life-long learner and multi-skilled global health professional. Dr Mabuza's mission is to improve health outcomes and to expand quality healthcare experiences amongst all groups of people and influence change and innovation.

www.ingramcontent.com/pod-product-compliance
Lightning Source LLC
Chambersburg PA
CBHW021749150726
47989CB00004B/1577